Intermittent Fasting For Women:

The Experts Guide to Losing 7 Lbs in 7 Days

TABLE OF CONTENTS

The Book At A Glance

In today's modern world, the accessibility to the immense universe of the World Wide Web has offered an extensive variety of trendy weight control programs and lifestyle changes, all promising great results. Popular programs include The Atkins Diet, Ketogenic Diet, Vegetarian Diet, Weight Watchers Diet, South Beach Diet, Zone Diet, and Intermittent Fasting.

But what is *'Fasting'* and why should you do it *intermittently*?

There are thousands of diet programs available today - some of them to enable individuals to shed pounds, some of them to enable to put on weight and some of them to simply help in developing a healthy and sustainable lifestyle. In the last few years, we have seen the shift from fast-food, upsize meals to the healthier choices of vegetables, fruits and, low-calorie eating programs that help people get stronger and healthier. This opens up a whole new era of nutrition-conscious individuals that focus on loving their body and helping them achieve the perfect lifestyle, which enables more people to see the better side of being healthy in the long run. As a matter of fact, in comparison to previous generations, a lot more individuals today are into exercising, increased involvement in sports activities leading some to say that millennials are more active and body conscious than their predecessors.

In this book, *Intermittent Fasting For Women: The Experts Guide to Losing 7 Lbs in 7 Days*, we will start off by introducing you to the world of Intermittent Fasting (IF) or what other people also call the *"8-hour diet"* (which you will later understand why they call this program the latter) and, the advantages of the fast and of course the disadvantages as well. The difference of this book from others that discuss IF is we give you the whole picture – we will define every single detail, the different schedules, and start you off on a bunch of recipes you can use to help you start off your fasting on a high note. FAQs are also included in the latter portion of the book, so that you won't have a hard time looking for answers elsewhere. As a bonus, we will include information, recipes, and more tidbits about Apple Cider Vinegar – what we consider our holy grail. In addition, we have also included a short subchapter of the popular diet programs out there and why intermittent fasting still tops all of them.

This book is guaranteed to help you understand fasting and why you should do it (if you haven't been yet) and help you maintain it. Here, you will understand why intermittent fasting deserves all the hype and why it's not just a one-off health and fitness trend. Is it healthy or does it even work? This book will be your complete guide about this lifestyle change and promises to leave you wanting to start fasting ASAP.

An Introduction to Fasting

A *diet* is defined as an eating routine that can likewise allude to the nourishment a person expends on every single day that affects the physical and psychological conditions of the human body. Though cliché, father of the Paleo diet, Jean Anthelme Brillat-Savarin once said, *"Tell me what you eat, and I will tell you what you are"*, and this quote has never been more evident in the past few years especially in this modern age where people have been introduced to cross cultural food from all walks of life.

Merriam and Webster's Dictionary defines *Intermittent* as the coming and going at intervals or something that is not continuous. It is described as something that lacks regularity in occurrence and examples consist of rain and employment.

Fasting, on the other hand, is defined as the abstinence of food and water intake for a certain period of time. It is previously well-associated with religious activities and spiritual observance.

Together, *Intermittent Fasting* is an eating pattern that alternates fasting and eating during the hours of the day. This type of program does not necessarily tell you what to eat and what not to eat, rather, it tells you when you should start eating and when to stop. Because of this, IF has seen a tremendous crowd following from all over the world, plus, it is backed by research and scientific studies.

Generally speaking, most people fast during the day without them knowing it. If you're someone who habitually skips breakfast, take up late lunches or sleep on dinner then technically, you're already fasting. To be honest, sleeping for 8 hours may also be considered fasting! Despite what other people may say, what's typically good about intermittent fasting is that it does not require you to count calories or skip carbs, rather, it just tells you that there is a schedule and a time for everything – eating and burning what you just ate. Intermittent fasting is giving your body enough time to burn all the food you have taken in and transform it into energy.

Some studies conclude that intermittent fasting can help you live longer while protecting you from diseases like diabetes, heart disease, Cancer, and Alzheimer's. Some may even go as far to consider that **intermittent fasting is so natural to man** that we have been doing it without us realizing.

There are a lot of different styles, schedules, and ways to do intermittent fasting. This book will introduce you to all of them to help you decide which one best suite your current lifestyle. But first, we will explain to you the 'Top 8 Diet Programs' and why you should just leave them alone and fast instead.

The Diet Mentality

So you've tried every single diet program offered out there and still, you're not near your goal weight. You've tried low-calorie, low-carb, and vegetarian programs but it's just so hard not to have that chocolate chip cookie or that delicious Bolognese pasta you've been craving two weeks now. You've tried exercising too but it's only good during the start and you're finding it hard to continue on because of your busy lifestyle. Or you have the time, and the gym is so near, but you're being held by budget constraints and family expenditures therefore annual memberships are really not your first priority. Eventually, you resort to looking for "the best diet program" out there that promises everyone great results. You may have seen it on the internet, or a friend just told you it worked on them, or you have seen so many people lose weight to this diet program so you're kind of sure it will work on you too. Sorry to break it to you but the honest deal about diet programs is that it will always depend on what your objectives are, and the type of body you have. What works on majority doesn't necessarily mean will work on you, and on the contrary, it doesn't also mean it won't.

According to Nordqvist, (2017) in an online article he published for website Medical News Today, he lists down the top diet programs with the biggest fan base. Combined with the research we performed to create this book, we list down the 'Top 8 Diet Programs' and what they are for to help you decide why Intermittent Fasting is the best choice for you.

1. **Atkins Diet:** One of the most popular diet programs available in the world today, the Atkins diet focuses on lowering insulin levels and keeping your carbohydrate intake low. While it helps you determine which carbs are healthy, the Atkins diet are not for those who needs a lot of energy to go through their day. And since there is a strict restriction on the type of food to eat, chances are, you'll be more tempted to binge-eating in the long haul.

2. **Ketogenic Diet:** initially designed as a therapeutic diet program for those with epilepsy, ketogenic diet aims to restrict calorie intake and focus on 75% fat and 20% protein, leaving the rest to carbohydrates. This diet program simply forces the body to use the fat and transform it into energy when all the carbohydrates in your body are gone. While this diet is easier to maintain compared to others, Ketogenic diet requires a huge body adjustment for 1-2 weeks which may leave the body weaker as your machinery tries to level with the program. Additionally, ketogenic diet is not recommended for those with high-blood pressure as this requires an individual to increase fat intake in replacement of carbohydrates.

3. **Vegetarian Diet:** According to (Stein, 2017), those who follow a strict all-vegetarian diet have a better control on their weight and are less likely to become obese. While this type of diet program promotes a healthier lifestyle because it only enables an individual to eat fruits and greens, it has a bigger potential for mineral and vitamin loss like iron and

Vitamin D; not to mention the lack in protein which the body also needs.

4. **Weight Watchers Diet:** Founded in 1963 by Jean Nidetch in New York, Weight Watchers diet program has been supported globally by celebrities and regular people alike. It works like a club or organization to help support each other by eating smarter and getting enough exercise. The main objective of the program is to control the portion of what you eat and encourages home cooking however, since it's a membership program, individuals on tight budgets are not advised to take on this program because of the high costs it may entail. Not to mention needing to participate in group meetings and weekly weigh-ins that may take a huge chunk off your schedule.

5. **South Beach Diet:** This popular diet program is celebrating its 15th anniversary this 2018 and has set a diet trend back in 2003 igniting the low-carb diet fad. What was initially designed for the prevention of heart disease, this diet promotes the consumption of food that contains heart-healthy unsaturated fats and is rich in fruits, vegetables and whole grains. But just like other low-carb diet programs, the South Beach Diet risks compromising vitamins and minerals that are essential for the body to function on a daily basis. Long term side effects may include rapid weight loss and liver abnormalities, probably because of the lack in scientific studies to support it.

6. **Zone Diet:** This diet uses the 40-30-30 ratio wherein an individual lowers their carbohydrate intake by only taking in 40% carbs, 30% fat and the

remaining 30% for protein. Though there is no banned food for this program and is notionally balanced in comparison to other diet programs, this eating pattern is not recommended for those with an active lifestyle. In addition, nutrition experts do not recommended this program to be taken for more than three consecutive months.

7. **Paleo Diet:** Also called the "cave-man diet", Paleo diet promotes eating like our ancestors by choosing to eat food without additives, preservatives and focusing on lean meat, seafood, fruits, non-starchy vegetables, seeds, and plant-based oils. Because of the limited food choices, people lose weight on this program however; it is extremely hard to follow because of the long list of restricted food. In addition to that, this program can get quite expensive because the allowed food is not too in demand and may be hard to find.

8. **DASH Diet:** According to (Frey, 2018) for the online article, *Pros and Cons of the DASH Diet*, this program has been voted the most favored diet program for the last few years. Also known as the Dietary Approaches to Stop Hypertension, this nutritional plans aims to encourage a high-fiber, low-fat diet to help reduce blood pressure. It consists of eating whole grains, fruits, and vegetables and eliminates the intake of carbonated drinks, fats, red meat, and sugary food. Though backed by studies from big organizations like the National Heart, Lung, and Blood Institute, this diet strictly follows a calorie intake program and may extremely difficult to maintain long term.

Why IF for Women?

Now that you have an idea about the other diet programs available out there, it is finally time to understand why intermittent fasting is best for women. While it swears by offering promising results and potential health benefits, like any other diet, it may also have some pros and cons.

The research conducted today explains that if done incorrectly, intermittent fasting may have an impact on women and their hormonal imbalance. In this book, we will discuss the best way to take on intermittent fasting and how you, as a woman, can maximize the benefits of going on a fast without risking the chances of endangering your chances of getting pregnant.

As stated by (Kollias, 2018), some women who have tried intermittent fasting have missed menstruation periods, early on-set menopause, cystic acne, and metabolism disturbances. Possibly, when the female body senses that the body is about to go on a fast, it rapidly increases the production of ghrelin and leptin which are hunger hormones. In turn, when the body gets the idea that the female body is starving, it tells the rest of the machinery to shut down, including the organs responsible for creating another human life form. The thing is, the female body does not know whether you're starving or just on a fast so it's best to get to know your body in any kind of diet program.

With all these challenges, you're probably wondering if it's still a good idea to go on a fast. Well the answer is – absolutely, yes! When done correctly, and learning more about your body and what works for you, intermittent fasting can help you reach your goal weight, achieve a healthy, well-balanced lifestyle without the risk of botching up your hormonal cycle.

Benefits of Fasting

In order to make a decision wholeheartedly, one has to look at both the pros and cons of any program or situation. Weighing up these options can help accelerate the basics these present, and writing up a list of pros and cons can help you approach your choice unbiasedly. In this book, *Intermittent Fasting For Women: The Experts Guide to Losing 7 Lbs. in 7 Days,* we do the listing for you so all you need to do is analyze the benefits and the side effects to know whether this is best suited for your lifestyle.

Overall, Intermittent Fasting promotes:

1. Weight Loss
2. Reduced Risk of Diabetes 2
3. Healthy Heart
4. Anti-Aging
5. Cancer Prevention
6. Less Inflammation and Oxidative Stress
7. Healthy Mind
8. Longer Life Span

Weight Loss

What tops off the benefits list of this program is of course, the weight loss (especially in belly fat). Because of the program's schedule of when to eat, this promotes less calorie intake which in turn also helps optimize hormones that are related to weight control.

The Fast State vs. the Fed State: During the *Fast State*, an individual is fasting and has not eaten anything at all. The most common is the 16/8 method wherein you are fasting for 16 hours therefore, will help you eat less. On the other hand, in the example mentioned, 8 hours is dedicated for eating and this is called the *Fed State*. Intermittent fasting is generally an advantageous method to limit calorie intake without the restrictions of other diets like low-carb or all-vegetarian. What this program promotes is for sthe body to be given enough time to burn all the food taken in and convert it to energy, therefore enabling you to get thinner and reduce belly fat in the process.

Reduced Risk of Diabetes 2

Diabetes 2, also known as Diabetes Mellitus Type 2 is a long-term metabolic disorder that is portrayed to a great degree of high glucose levels, insulin resistance and lack thereof. When an individual is intermittently fasting, it allows the body to take a break and pushes the body to use up all its sugar stores. This process helps insulin levels drop and makes the machinery become sensitive and responsive to insulin once again.

Healthy Heart

The World Heart Federation (WHF) established World Heart Day in 2009 to help fight the world's biggest killer – cardiovascular disease (CVD) or simply known as heart disease. Based on the studies done for intermittent fasting, results have shown that overall blood pressure has improved, cholesterol and triglycerides and blood sugar markers have gone down therefore promoting a healthier heart.

Anti-Aging

According to (Adorante, 2017) for W Magazine's September 2017 issue, holistic nutritionist to the stars Kelly LeVeque states that she would rather have her celebrity clients on an intermittent fasting program than any other because it helps with slow down the aging process as compared to eating every 3-4 hours. Intermittent fasting helps the body's autophagy process and promote cellular repair. When your cells have the ability to repair quickly, it has a higher chance of slowing down the process of aging.

Cancer Prevention

According to (Dr. David Jockers DC, 2016), he has recommended intermittent fasting to Cancer patients and subsequently, to the prevention of the mentioned disease. He calls the fed state the *'Building Phase'* wherein the body fills up the machinery through the food intake and builds up all necessary vitamins and minerals it needs during the day. Diversely, the doctor calls the fast state the 'Cleansing Phase' where the body cleanses and transforms the minerals into energy that's why it is so important to have a longer period of cleansing. When the body is given enough time to cleanse and detoxify, the more time it has to kill off viruses in your body, potentially including cancer cells.

Less Inflammation & Oxidative Stress

Inflammation isn't constantly decent or constantly awful sort of reaction. We encounter inflammation when our body is endeavoring to recuperate itself, yet when it goes on for extensive stretches of time, negative wellbeing impacts happen and our bodies naturally give in to disease.

Based on multiple research studies, excessive inflammation may cause many types of disorders in the body including but not limited to dementia, Alzheimer's, diabetes, obesity and many more. On the positive side of things, intermittent fasting helps reduce the body's inflammation therefore helping keep the machinery from chronic diseases.

Autophagy is a physiological process of the body that destroys old or damaged cells in order to process new cells. When old and damaged cells remain for longer periods in the body, inflammation starts. Intermittent fasting helps boost the process of autophagy to help the body detoxify itself therefore reducing inflammation.

Healthy Mind

According to a study conducted by esteemed John Hopkins professor, Dr. Mark Mattson, intermittent fasting has shown tremendous increase of neurogenesis when done systematically. Neurogenesis is the natural process of the brain to produce new nerve cells. In an active process, neurogenesis conducts an active production of neurons, and, other stem cells. He asserts that intermittent fasting bolsters brain power therefore can boost brain performance, mood, and memory among others.

Longer Life Span

In a new study conducted by Harvard, it shows how intermittent fasting helps an individual achieve a longer life span. Because of the many benefits of intermittent fasting to the body, it prevents the individual from acquiring chronic diseases therefore preserving the body and turning up the safety walls of the machinery. In addition to this, intermittent fasting also helps alter mitochondrial processes in the body. Mitochondria are the cell's inner battery operators and are prominently in charge of super-charging the cells. Senior author to the study, William Mair says that intermittent fasting helps manipulate the mitochondria into staying on a "youthful" state.

Side-Effects of Fasting

As you have red, there are numerous benefits to intermittent fasting including weight loss, cancer prevention, healthy mind and heart, and prevention of chronic diseases. By this time, you may be convinced to try it but this book aims to give you all the details associated with intermittent fasting, including the not-so-awesome side affects you may experience especially in the beginning.

Note: Before you start any kind of diet plan, make sure to check with your doctor first. And don't forget to listen to your body.

1. Hunger Pangs
2. Persistent Cravings
3. Low Energy Levels
4. Headaches, Migraines, and Flu
5. Irritability
6. Bloating and Constipation or Diarrhea
7. Overeating

Hunger Pangs

Your body has been used to eating more than 6x daily with no schedule therefore at most times, your body kind of expects food. The first few days of your fast are the most critical and challenging because this is when the hormone ghrelin is most active. Also known as the "hunger hormone", ghrelins are responsible to send signals to your brain when it comes to eating. A hormone produced in the human's gut, it travels through the bloodstreams and tells the brain that it is hungry and that it should look for food. This hunger signals usually peak during regular meal times – breakfast, lunch, dinner or even snack time, depending on your regular food intake. The first five days will be really challenging as you will be tempted to seek out food and the only way to combat this is your strong willpower. After these, your body will well adjust to the window hours and soon enough, you won't feel hungry at all.

According to fitness sensation Mario Tomic, one of the best ways to combat hunger pangs is to drink water. He states that most of the time, hunger signals can be very misleading because the ghrelins tell your brain you're hungry but truth is, you might just be thirsty. During the fast period or at any point you feel incredibly hungry, it would be best to load up on water, tea or coffee. He even suggests that brushing your teeth during these times would help lessen the hunger signals. Lastly, Tomic advises that in order for each person to truly control their hunger hormones, they must get enough sleep. Shortened sleep time is often associated with increased levels of hunger, as it tries to get more energy from the food intake.

Persistent Cravings

During the fast period, your body signals the brain to think about food a lot since you're not getting it. Because of this, you start thinking about all the good food and your cravings starts – pizza, pasta, ice cream, steak, name it, it'll come up. The craving for sweets and carbohydrates also increases because the body is starting to look for the glucose hit it has been getting before the fast. According to (Crain, 2015) for the magazine, Women's Health, she advises that when the cravings start to sip in, try going for a walk, play a video game, sip water or tea, or just take a break and start thinking of something else. Just like the hunger pangs, it will be extremely hard during the first few days but hang on to your goals and you'll eventually get over it.

Low Energy Levels

When your body starts to shift from eating a lot to fasting on a schedule, the body starts to feel a little sluggish and tired. During the first few days, beg away from heavy tasks, lifting or rigor exercise activities. Instead, take a nap, try to relax a little so that your body doesn't collapse with the sudden adjustment to food intake.

Headaches, Migraines, Flu

Headaches are a pretty common side effect when there is a lifestyle change or a change in diet. Most people complain about frequent bursts of headaches while some have them all throughout the new process. Some people have elevated types of headaches and get migraines for hours during the first few days. Others have reported that they also get down with the flu once they fast and this some ways your body tells you they are adjusting. One of the best ways to cure the headache or migraine is to load up on water. And if the symptoms persist, it would be best to check with your doctor.

Irritability

People who are hungry are generally irritable. No one wants to feel hungry but when you start to fast, you will feel hungry all the time during the first few days. When you start feeling cranky, think of the happy things that make you a little less irritable or look forward to the meals you're going to take during your fed state.

Bloating, Constipation or Diarrhea

Bloating can usually be felt once you start eating after a long fast. Sometimes, it would make you feel uncomfortably full. Not getting your usual amount of food may also make you constipated or the other way around – have Diarrhea. This is due to the huge change your body is making and the best way to address this is again, water! Drink up on lots of water – more than what you usually take. This will be your body's refuge.

Overeating

Some people tend to overeat during the start of their fasting because, well, you can basically eat anything during your fed state. This is partially true. Even if you're allowed to eat anything in general, that doesn't necessarily mean you eat 10x more than what you previously take in. of course you still need to watch out for the food you take in, especially if you want t results fast.

Fasting Schedules

There are multiple ways to do intermittent fasting. This book will give you a guide on the most popular methods or schedules that have been backed up by science. As a friendly reminder, it would be best to contact your doctor or nutritionist for questions regarding your meal plan, your health or any symptoms you may experience during the fast. Also remember that the body is different from one person to another therefore, a person's results may not be the same for another.

The concept of losing weight is very simple: you should be able to burn off more calories than the ones you take in. Going on diet programs is not only a one-off process but a long-term method that will take perseverance, hard work and a big amount of willpower.

It's important that in the event that you fully decide to go on intermittent fasting, it is best to remember that to begin with, perceive that the main part of a weight loss program is the amount of food you take in, not the amount of exercise you associate with. Though exercise plays a crucial role in the weight loss journey, it basically just helps you stay in shape, build and safeguard muscles tissue, expanding perseverance, and aids in burning the calories you took in.

Having a plan for your intermittent fasting will determine how successful you will be in achieving your goal. This chapter focuses on the different types of methods, and schedules available for intermittent fasting so that you will have a better understanding of the program to help you decide which one is best suited for your body. Knowing the pros and cons of each method will determine how you may want to incorporate this program into your current lifestyle.

Being a woman is not an easy feat but women who have discipline and have set their eyes on a goal can achieve anything.

Daily Intermittent Fasting (16:8 Plan)

16 Hours Fasted

8 Hours Fed

The most popular amongst all the schedules of intermittent fasting, the daily intermittent fasting otherwise also known as the Leangains Method was popularized by nutritional consultant and personal trainer, Martin Berkhan. And because this schedule is done every day, it's the easiest to get into the habit of eating on this particular schedule. Fasting for 16 long hours of the day and allowing your body a solitary eight-hour window for eating could be a decent choice for beginners.

Who is it for? Individuals who would like to achieve and maintain a lean physique. This may also be taken by those who would like to lose weight

How to Do It? Fast for 16 hours and eat for 8 hours on the daily. What's great about this program is that it lets you do it when your schedule permits you to. The best way to do your fast according to the expert himself is to place a large chunk of the 16 hours while you're sleeping so you won't notice time slipping.

Alternate Day Intermittent Fasting

24 Hours Fed

24 Hours Fast

This method is as simple as it gets: fast every other day. Alternate fasting lets you eat whatever you want for 24 hours and for the next 24 hours, go on a strict low-calorie diet, suggestively 600 calories for men and 500 calories for women.

Who is it for? Individuals who have been fasting for more than a year and have adjusted their machineries to the schedules and side-effects of fasting can try this method. This is not recommended for beginners as a full 24 hour fast may be too extreme. The aim of this fast is to basically restrict the calories and lose weight.

How to Do It? Fast for 16 hours and eat for 8 hours on the daily. What's great about this program is that it lets you do it when your schedule permits you to. The best way to do your fast according to the expert himself is to place a large chunk of the 16 hours while you're sleeping so you won't notice time slipping.

The Warrior Fast

20 Hours Fasted

4 Hours Fed

One of the first methods introduced in intermittent fasting, the Warrior Diet was influenced by ancient war societies of Sparta and Rome. Popularized by Ori Hofmekler, a fitness expert, this method allows you to eat fruits and vegetables during the day and eat one huge meal at night. He invented this schedule back in 2001 after serving with the Israeli Special Forces. To simply put it, you're supposed to fast for 20 hours and eat big at night for a window of 4 hours. If you adapt to the diet Hofmekler advises, your body will be pushed to burn the fat it takes in for fuel.

Who is it for? The Warrior Diet is considered a holistic approach kind of diet as it requires a good exercise regimen to support the method. This diet is recommended for those who are looking to build more muscle mass and gain survivor instincts.

How to Do It? Fast for 20 hours, eating only light fruits, vegetables and lots of water. At night, you may eat 1 heavy meal during the 4 hour window.

Eat-Stop-Eat (1/6 Fast Plan)

1 Day Fasted

6 Days Fed

Fast for 24 Hours Once or Twice a Week

This method, popularized by fitness guru Brad Pilon, allows you to fast 1-2 times per week and eat normally for the remaining days. Because you eat regularly for 6 days and only fast for 1-2 days, some people find this method easier to follow. The reason behind Pilon's popular method is because he believes that people tend to get obsessed with food once they fast "too much", leaving them overeating once they're off the fasting period. During your fasting days, Pilon suggests to eat 500-600 calories per day or light calorie meals to keep the pounds away but still be able to eat whatever you want on other days. Bottom-line is, you eat regularly and fast for 24 hours. What's great about this method is that it has been studied scientifically by several notable research institutions and has concluded this schedule as one of the most effective methods to lose weight. Some studies even state that this type of method is more effective than fasting every day.

Who is it for? Individuals who would like to achieve and maintain a lean physique and those who want to build more muscle.

How to Do It? Generally, fast for 1 day and feed for 6 days a week. What makes this method work is because it's easier to follow for the long term. This schedule works for most individuals who want to get lean because the body can easily handle low calorie plans every once in a while without botching up the body's regular metabolism.

The 5:2 Diet (24-Hour Fast)

5 Days Fed

2 Days Fast 500-600 Calories/Day

The 5:2 diet schedule, popularized by Dr. Michael Mosley, journalist and medic allows you to eat what you want for five days a week and fast for your chosen two days. However, the recommend calorie intakes on fasting days are 600 calories for men and 500 for women.

Who is it for? Also called the "Fast Diet", this intermittent fasting schedule is best for those who would like to lose weight and improve health.

How to Do It? Fast for 2 days during the week, taking in food amounting to 500-600 calories a day only. The rest of the days (5), you can generally eat anything you want. A 500-calorie meal plan consists of 1 large boiled egg for breakfast, 1 cup of blackberries for lunch accompanied by 4 oz. of grilled salmon, and 1/3 cup of green beans with 1/3 cup of quinoa for dinner.

7 Day Meal Plans to Help You Start

You've learned everything about intermittent fasting including the benefits, side-effects, and the schedule. This time, you want to maximize the results and get on a proper meal plan to kick of your new lifestyle. Well, fret not – this book has got you covered.

Here is an outline of your first 7 days to help you get in the game and lose 7 lbs. in 7 days. Remember to check with your doctor or nutritionist especially for special cases.

Day OneDay Two

Day Three

Day Four

Day Five

Day Six

Day Seven

	Monday	Tues	Wed	Thurs	Fri	Sat	Sun
Breakfast	1 cup Oatmeal and 1/2 sliced Banana	Egg White Omelet with Mushrooms Spinach Bell Pepper 1 slice of Whole Grain Toast or 1/2 cup Fruit	1 Non-fat Greek Yogurt and 1 Tbsp. Silvered Almonds	1 Medium Sweet Potato and 1/4 cup Black Beans	1 Glass Smoothie With unsweetened Vanilla or Chocolate Protein powder Unsweetened Almond Milk on Shaved Ice	1/2 cup Fiber-rich Cereal 1 cup light Soy Milk	2 slices Whole Wheat Bread 1 Tbsp. Natural Peanut Butter 2 Tsp. Jam 1 Cup Skim Milk
Dinner	1 cup Quinoa and Spinach + 4 oz. Pan-Seared Salmon	4 oz. Chicken Breast 1 cup Spaghetti Squash 1/2 cup Broccoli 1/2 cup Cauliflower with Marinara Sauce	Large Salad 3 oz. Chicken Breast 1 Tbsp Silvered Almonds 1/4 cup grapefruit or orange slices	Portobello Mushroom Grilled or Burger Whole Wheat Sandwich 1/2 cup sweet potato	2 oz. Black Bean Pasta with Spinach, Mushrooms, Bell pepper, Zucchini	3 oz. Pan Roasted Tilapia with Mediterranean Tomato Sauce 1/2 cup Quinoa 1 cup Steamed Camote	1 Cup Vegetable Soup 3 oz. Turkey 2 Small Apple Slices 2 Slices Whole Wheat Bread 1 Cup Skim Milk
Snacks				Water, Tea, Coffee			

The Miraculous Apple Cider Vinegar

Apple Cider Vinegar (ACV) is a type of vinegar that is made from apples, sugar, and yeast. What was once used only for salad dressings and preservatives, apple cider vinegar has come a long way since the 1970s when folks started using this as a go-to home remedy to treat anything from sore throat to infection prevention. One of the benefits apple cider vinegar is known for is its sterling ability to help people lose weight. In the recent years, apple cider vinegar has taken the spotlight topping off other natural remedies like tea tree oil, and other well-known natural helpers. But first, let's take a closer look at what this potion is all about to determine what we can use it for, of course besides an aid for weight loss.

Composition

Made up of apple juice, yeast is added to the solution to make the fruit sugar alcoholic. This process is otherwise known as fermentation. After which, the bacteria found in the juice turns the alcohol into acetic acid, or vinegar.

Benefits

1. **Soothes Sore Throat** – most germs can't make due in the acidic condition vinegar has therefore apple cider vinegar may be used to relieve yourself from the itchy, sore throat.

2. Mix ¼ glass of apple cider vinegar w/ ¼ cup of warm water and gargle every hour.

3. **Lowers Cholesterol, Prevents Obesity and Helps You Lose Weight** – a Japanese study found that half an ounce of apple cider vinegar drank per day lowers cholesterol levels. And because the composition of the apple cide vinegar contains acetic acid, this helps suppress your appetite, reduce water retention and curbs your metabolism – SWEET.

4. **Helps Clear Stuffy Nose Due to Colds** – the oldest trick in the book, mixing 2 Tbsps. Of apple cider vinegar to a glass of warm water can help relieve you of a stuffy nose. This is because apple cider vinegar contains potassium (yes, the same one found in bananas!) which is known to effectively thin out mucus.

5. **Helps Give You Shiny, Bouncy Hair, and Gets Rid of the Dandruff** – Because apple cider vinegar helps with the pH levels of the skin, it can also help with the skin on head or also known as the scalp. It basically makes bacteria go away because the yeast prevents it to grow. Spritz on your scalp and let it sit on your hair like a conditioner for 15 minutes to an hour. Doing this twice a week can help achieve maximum results.

6. **Helps Clear Acne** – a lot of people use apple cider vinegar as an organic toner as its antibacterial properties can help keep acne under control while maintaining the pH balance of your skin.

7. **Boosts Energy** – there are a ton of amino acids found in apple cider vinegar and this can help with keeping your shutters open. And because it contains potassium and enzymes, it can help you keep up

with your busy schedule. Mix a tablespoon to a glass of water and you're ready to go.

8. **Controls Blood Sugar** – a study conducted by the Arizona State University found that people who were resistant to insulin drank a mix of apple cider vinegar and water had shown decreases blood sugar levels. This may be due to the antiglycemic effect of the vinegar.

Apple Cider for Weight Loss

As indicated in one of the studies performed, 1 or 2 tablespoons of apple cider vinegar to your eating routine can enable you to get in shape. It can likewise diminish your muscle to fat ratio; influence you to lose belly fat and abatement your blood triglycerides. What makes apple cider vinegar is its ability to curb the appetite to further aid in weight loss programs. Apple cider vinegar can help you trick your tummy to think it's full. A study by dietician Erin Palinski-Wade, RD, CDE suggests that people who consume apple cider vinegar after a meal have a less chance of feeling hungry sooner. In addition, acetic acid is considered a natural appetite suppressant therefore helps in curbing the appetite.

1. Morning Detox Drink

   1 Tbsp. of Apple Cider Vinegar

   1 Tbsp. of Lemon Juice

   1 Tbsp. of Raw or Organic Honey

   1 Tsp. of Grated Ginger

   2 oz. of Water

   Mix all of the ingredients together; may be served cold, warm or hot.

   Begin your day with a glass of the invigorating apple cider vinegar solution and stay re-energized all throughout the day. This pick-me-up concoction has a tasty sweet and tart flavor that also works with a sugar-loaded natural product juices .The blend of cinnamon and ginger improves the kinds of the drink while the nectar adjusts the solid taste of the apple juice vinegar to make it more suitable to the taste.

   Benefits of Apple – The dissolvable fiber gelatin found in apple has the ability to impact weight reduction. Gelatin retains water and structures a gel-like mass in the stomach and small digestive tract that backs off processing and expands satiety. It gives enough time to the stomach receptors to flag the cerebrum that the stomach is full and thus the mind triggers the arrival of hormones that builds the feeling of satiety. Gelatin likewise helps glucose direction that diminishes the arrival of insulin in blood.

Nectar – Honey not just goes about as a characteristic sweetener that improves the essence of the drink, yet in addition advances weight reduction by boosting body digestion. It additionally has the capacity to assemble put away fat and make it accessible as a fuel for doing your everyday exercises.

2. Evening Detox Mix

2 Tsp. Apple Cider Vinegar

2 Tbsp. Lemon Juice

1 Tsp. Honey

1 Tsp. Ground Cinnamon

1 Cup Hot Water

End your tiring day with this heavenly apple cider vinegar drink that tastes nearly in the same class as crusty fruit-filled treat that can help you relax after a long and tiring day. The mouth-watering kinds of honey, cinnamon, and a cup of warm water can totally conceal the solid kinds of the vinegar and make it a solitary drink.

Benefits of Cinnamon – This delightful zest is helpful for weight reduction in a few different ways. Initially, cinnamon controls insulin levels in the body and manage blood glucose levels and aims to burn excess fat especially in the belly. Also, it accelerates digestion with the goal that your body consumes more calories notwithstanding when it is very still. Thirdly, it stifles hunger by backing off the procedure of entry of sustenance through the digestion tracts which encourages you to feel full for a more extended timeframe.

3. Apple Cider Vinegar Fat Burning Mix

1 Tbsp. Apple Cider Vinegar

1 Tbsp. Lemon Juice

1 Tbsp. Raw, Organic Honey

1 Tsp. Cayenne Powder

Mix all ingredients together and drink 30 mins before each meal

This apple cider vinegar detox drink comes straight from Dr. Hatchet and it comprises of every single normal fixing. This compelling detox drink serves to gets and flushes out poisons from the body, help vitality, advance fat and battles infections. The blend of lemon juice and cayenne gives a pleasant exquisite and tart taste to the drink while cinnamon adds an invigorating flavor to it.

Benefits of Cayenne – Capsaicin, the principle dynamic fixing present in cayenne pepper is a thermogenic synthetic that velocities up your digestion and advances speedier calorie consume. Research demonstrates that cayenne pepper can expand general digestion by very nearly 25%. It likewise helps in checking craving with the goal that you include exhaust calories by nibbling unfortunate nourishments.

4. Green Tea and Apple Cider Vinegar

1 Green Tea bag (steep in hot water and remove)

1 Tbsp. Apple Cider Vinegar

1 Tsp. Honey

This mitigating and reviving apple juice vinegar green tea is even more unwinding refreshment as opposed to a detox drink. This apple juice vinegar drink is particularly valuable for alleviating swelling and fart. It likewise gives a moment increase in vitality and when taken between dinners it holds your craving in line and averts unaware eating. The cool and crisp kinds of the green tea impeccably adjust the solid kind of the apple juice vinegar.

Green tea – Green is the most beneficial refreshment on the planet stuffed with cancer prevention agents and bioactive substances that assistance in getting more fit. EGCG a catching found in green tea has the ability to support digestion so your body consumes calories notwithstanding when it is very still. EGCG likewise has the ability to prepare fat from the fat cells and make them accessible for use as vitality by the muscle cells.

5. Apple Cider and Pineapple Smoothie

1 cup Pineapples slices

1 Cup Water

2 Tbsp. Apple Cider Vinegar

1 Tbsp. Honey

Blend all ingredients together in a blender until smooth. Serve.

Eager to lay off the coffee? This morning concoction will help you do just that. Supplant your morning espresso with this tasty and power-stuffed apple juice vinegar drink and get a moment increase in energy to kick begin your morning. It helps in reinforcing the insusceptible framework while boosting digestion with the goal that your body keeps on consuming calories even very still. The pineapple squeeze and lime juice cooperate to give a decent tart taste to the drink, while the nectar adds a smooth sweetness to it.

Benefits of Pineapple – Enzyme bromelain found in pine apple eases aggravation and advance assimilation – both of which help in weight reduction. The vast majority of us are uninformed of the way that irritation is one of the main sources of weight pick up. Bromelain battle and diminish irritation so hormone leptin can work all the more productively to control body weight. Bromelain diminishes stomach related issues, for example, swelling, gas and crabby inside disorder, which thusly helps the body to separate sustenance and retain the supplements all the more viably. Every one of these things positively affects your digestion rate.

6. Cranberry Juice Drink

1 tablespoon of apple cider vinegar

¾ cup of water

½ cup of cranberry juice

Splash of lime juice

Add all the ingredients in a bowl of hot water. Stir properly. Pour into a glass and drink. Add extra lime juice for more sweetness.

Looking for something refreshing during the afternoon? This concoction can also be substituted for a mocktail drink, wherein the refreshing flavors of cranberry juice and lime dilute the sour taste of vinegar.

Benefits of Cranberry - Cranberries are water-gathered organic products. They are stuffed with supplements to enable your body to avert diseases and lift general wellbeing. When paired with apple cider vinegar, this concoction will make a power-packed anti-oxidant drink that will surely help you shed off those pounds in no time.

Bonus Recipes

Apple Cider Vinegar Foot Soak

> 5 Cups of Apple Cider Vinegar
>
> 1 Gallon Warm Water
>
> 1 Large Bowl for Soak
>
>> Add 5 cups of apple cider vinegar to 1 gallon of warm water in a large bowl. Stir and soak the both feet in this mix for 15 minutes. After which, take out feet and pat dry. Do this twice weekly to relieve foot pain and cramps especially for women who love wearing heels.

Apple Cider Vinegar Salad Dressing

> Olive Oil
>
> Apple Cider Vinegar
>
> Dijon Mustard
>
> Sea Salt
>
> Garlic
>
> Pepper
>
> Mix ingredients together in a bowl. Add salt and pepper to taste.

Making Intermittent Fasting Your New Lifestyle

Along the line, you've probably heard that changing your diet is not just a method or process that takes a few months or a year. To be honest, it's a complete overhaul of your lifestyle. Intermittent fasting is no different and requires you to adapt into this new lifestyle. Once you've decided to take the daily intermittent fasting that allows you to eat for 8 hours and fast for 16 hours, you would need to do this every single day. You don't stop because you're near your goal; you stop because it's enough. It's enough that you're healthy and in high spirits. Your body is going to thank you for it, for being patient and willing to go the distance only to take care of it.

As a final word from this book, here is a final list of the things to help you go forth with your weight loss and achieve a healthy mind, body, and heart. If anything, individuals who "count calories" tend to put on more weight after some time, and studies demonstrate that eating less junk food is a steady indicator of future weight pick up. Rather than starting to eat less, make it your objective to wind up a more beneficial, more joyful and fitter individual. Don't diet, eat healthy.

1. **Drink LOTS of Water** - Drinking 0.5 liters of water may build the measure of calories consumed for no less than 60 minutes. A few examinations demonstrate this can prompt unassuming weight reduction. Since water is normally sans calorie, it is by and large connected with diminished calorie

consumption. This is for the most part since you at that point drink water rather than different refreshments, which are regularly high in calories and sugar. Observational investigations have demonstrated that individuals who drink for the most part water have up to a 9% bring down calorie admission, by and large. Drinking water may likewise help forestall long haul weight pick up. All in all, the normal individual increases around 1.45 kg at regular intervals.

2. **Drink Green Tea** - The bioactive substances in the tea leaves break down in the water and make it into the last drink. When you drink some quality tea, you're really getting a lot of helpful substances with strong organic impacts.

3. The best known about these is caffeine. Some green tea contains significantly less caffeine than some espresso , yet at the same time enough to have a mellow impact.. Caffeine is an outstanding stimulant that has been appeared to help fat consuming and enhance practice execution in various examinations. In any case, where green tea truly sparkles is in its enormous scope of cancer prevention agents... being stacked with intense cell reinforcements called catechins. The most critical of these is EGCG, a substance that can help digestion.

4. **Cut back on the Sugar** – Excessive soda drinking represents in excess of a fourth of all beverages devoured inside the United States. Beginning at child age, youngsters are drinking soda and adding more sugar to their bodies than treats, sweet and frozen yogurt joined. Alongside this, caffeine may also be

seen as a major culprit and these two synthetics are the ideal tempest for a deep rooted dependence on carbonated beverages. Once you learn to cut back on the soda, you start losing interest in sweet and sugary drinks or food in particular. Evaluations demonstrate that two jars or glasses of soda every day adds roughly 24 to 35 pounds of fat for each year, contingent upon body estimate, age, propensities, and so on.. A few people have revealed that by surrendering two jars of soda for each day, without work out, they lost 20 pounds in a half year. Include work out, lessen other sugar admission, eat more foods grown from the ground, include high water utilization and you could be prepared to fit into those pants inside a month and a half. Be that as it may, if removing pop inside and out is excessively troublesome, you could supplant one soda for each day with water.

5. **Eat Less Carbs** – Many times it has been mentioned in the book that one of the benefits of intermittent fasting is the fact that you can eat anything during your fed state. But it doesn't mean you can just eat carbs on carbs on carbs during your 8 hour window. Practice portion control. Eat less of the carbs and load up on the fiber and the protein.

6. **Use Smaller Plates** – one way of tricking the mind that it's full is to use smaller plates. Studies show that those individuals who eat on a smaller plate tend to signal their brain to stop eating since they've already consumed what's on the plate. Your mind works a similar way and feels fulfilled when you eat a little

plate brimming with food contrasted with a vast plate with a similar sum.

7. **Move, move, and move** - Devouring fewer calories and incorporating less fat in your eating regimen is important to shed pounds. Including exercise builds the quantity of calories you consume with the goal that you speed your weight reduction. A few people say that activity expands their yearning. In any case, practice pulls put away calories in the types of glucose and fat out of tissues with the goal that blood glucose levels remain even and you don't feel hungry.

8. The more calories you consume over the sum that your body needs to keep up its present weight, the more noteworthy your weight reduction. That is the reason adding activity to your diminished calorie design accelerates your weight reduction endeavors. Another way that activity consumes calories is by expanding your metabolic rate. What's more, practice causes you to lose fat yet not muscle, which decides how quick or moderate your body consumes calories. Fat is generally latent, however muscle is dynamic and necessities vitality to look after itself. So the more muscle you have, the more calories your body needs.

9. **Chew More Slowly** - Your hunger and calorie admission is generally controlled by hormones. Typically subsequent to eating, your gut stifles a hormone called ghrelin, which controls hunger. These hormones transfer a message to the mind, telling it that you've eaten and that food is being ingested. This diminishes craving, influences you to

feel full, and encourages you quit eating. Strangely, this procedure takes around 20 minutes, so backing off gives your cerebrum the time it needs to get these signs and tells your mind you're full.

Safety and Precautions of Intermittent Fasting

Intermittent fasting is just abandoning sustenance for a more drawn out timeframe than you're utilized to. The excellence is that the period of time can shift from individual to individual, somewhere in the range of 16 hours to 24 hours and the measure of long stretches of irregular fasting can fluctuate also. Some benefits of intermittent fasting incorporate weight reduction, insulin affectability, averting mind maturing and expanding cell vitality generation. The mix of both calorie confinement and discontinuous fasting ended up being very successful for diminishing weight and bringing down the danger of cardiovascular illness in one examination.

Every one of these advantages accompanies a few safety measures nonetheless. As I would like to think, irregular fasting should be done warily and after some primer work on the body. For example, going from a standard American eating regimen to cutting calories and fasting is likely not the best method to shed pounds or empower ideal wellbeing. Preceding consolidating discontinuous fasting it is essential to comprehend your glucose levels and how your body responds to pressure.

At the point when your glucose levels drop significantly, cortisol (a pressure hormone) raises, which thus causes the glucose to lift keeping in mind the end goal to standardize the precariousness. This is regularly something you need to maintain a strategic distance from, as we in a perfect world would prefer not to do things that fundamentally increment cortisol generation. This implies irregular fasting can really make more weight on the body by fluctuating glucose levels too significantly. So above all else, before driving straight into discontinuous fasting or calorie confinement we would first pick up control of glucose levels and make a solid association with push. This can be hard for individuals and it can require a long investment before that trust is made. Thus, returning to the possibility that we have to eat each 2-3 hours. This is the manner by which trust is made with the body.

The initial step is to adjust your proportion of proteins, fats and carbs while diminishing straightforward sugars and basic starches.

Eat inside an hour and a half of waking and dependably have a high protein breakfast, parity your dinners with loads of vegetables, great protein and sound fats. Help your body diminish cortisol by unwinding, working out, and resting soundly. When this soundness is made inside the establishment of your body then you can push ahead into calorie confinement and irregular fasting and receive every one of the rewards. Discontinuous fasting and calorie confinement can have astounding advantages for the body as we've seen, for example, weight reduction, insulin affectability and ideal cell work however take note of that it can likewise make undesirable weight on the body in the event that you have not set aside the opportunity to assemble an appropriate establishment.

Always remember to proceed with caution. If you are sick, diagnosed with any type of sickness, please consult your doctor, your nutritionist or dietician. They are the experts and they know your body and what works for you.

The mind-body association has for some time been built up, and a large portion of us can fold our heads over the physical weaknesses of mental pressure. I'm going above and beyond to state that the body and soul are inseparably interlaced. I'm discussing care, your profound prosperity, and the peace that originates from knowing and adoring yourself profoundly. Figure your body isn't getting on those signs? Matters of the spirit rapidly progress toward becoming issues of the body and the other way around. Tuning in to and for the most part respecting your body regularly implies completing an enthusiastic registration. How does your sensory system respond to half a month of consecutive social commitment? Is it accurate to say that you are feeling energized and engaged where you're at, or completely overpowered? Ask and tune in. The data you get will enable you to recognize what feels ideal from what feels right, at the present time. Being profoundly mindful of your body and ready to comprehend things like your yearning signs, how your feelings drive your development and eating choices, and how stretch shows in your body is exceedingly profitable.

Truth be told, it's one of the contrasts between individuals who battle with eating regimen and exercise as long as they can remember, and individuals who build up a sound association with their bodies, sustenance and wellness. The effective people have assembled the abilities, through training, that enable them to be careful, focus on their feelings, and tune into their body's signs. Luckily, the aptitude of aggregating self-information — what we may call tuning in to your body and realizing what works for you — is only that, an expertise

FAQ's of Intermittent Fasting

1. What is intermittent fasting?

Answer: It is an eating pattern that alternates fasting and eating during the hours of the day. This type of program does not necessarily tell you what to eat and what not to eat, rather, it tells you when you should start eating and when to stop.

2. Who Is Intermittent Fasting For?

Answer: It is generally for anyone who wants to lose weight, and improve their healthy habits. It is recommended for people who want to live longer and healthier.

3. Is There A Proper Age To Start Fasting?

Answer: People have been known to fast since ancient times without people realizing they're already fasting so it should be fine. However, to be on the safe side of things, it would be better to consult your dietician, physician, and your nutritionist if you're below legal age.

4. Does intermittent fasting have a schedule or pattern?

Answer: Yes, there are multiple types of intermittent fasting method but the popular ones are: Daily Intermittent Fasting, Alternate Day Intermittent Fasting, The Warrior Fast, Eat-Stop-Eat, and The 5:2 Diet.

5. Won't intermittent fasting make me hungry?

Answer: During the first few days of the fast, you will experience a lot of hunger pangs, and food cravings. However, once your body has adjusted to the schedule and the fast, you will slowly overcome these hurdles and achieve your goal.

6. I have work during the day and I tend to eat while at work. How will this work for me?

Answer: One of the best things about intermittent fasting is that it does not generally tell you what to eat. With the different schedules available, it won't be hard to find the one that best fits your lifestyle, and your schedule.

7. Can I add cream or milk to my coffee?

Answer: It's actually up to you. But for ultimate results, black coffee is recommended.

8. Can I still workout even when I'm fasting?

Answer: Exercise is encouraged in any kind of program but rigorous and extensive exercise is not recommended if you're trying this out for the first time.

9. Is intermittent fasting safe for women?

Answer: This is the greatest territory of contention when it comes to intermittent fasting. The individuals who alert ladies against intermittent fasting say that it has great impacts against fertility and some studies have shown it to be true. However, they do not include the facts of the study where women who have experience fertility challenges after a fast practice an alternate kind of fast where do not eat anything for a full 24 hours. While it is recommended for some, women (and even men) still have to check with their physician whether it would be good for them to fast and which method would greatly benefit them.

Just a precaution though that intermittent fasting is not safe for pregnant women or women with certain diagnosis. It is best to check with your doctor before committing to any fasting or diet program.

10. Why is intermittent fasting effective?

Answer: Because it allows the body enough time to cleanse, the body is able to cope up with the different kinds of stresses thrown at it. Because of this, he body is able to heal itself and regenerate new cells.

Final Word

Intermittent fasting, like any other diet or weight loss program requires a huge amount of willpower and determination to complete. If you're the type to easily give up if things get a little hard then this may not be the right method for you. But if you're that woman who's tired of being unhealthy and instead be that someone who wants to start getting better physically, then it's about time you start this fitness journey.

The fitness industry is full of myths and false promises. Some promise the world on a scale of losing 20 lbs. in 5 days but fail to let on the promise. People are advised to do all sorts of nasty and out-of-this-world things for the sake of getting leaner, fit, and sexy but they don't explain the whole process. There has been a pendulum of all sorts of programs from low carb, no carb, low fat, no fat, all-veggie diet and other kinds of methods that promise the sun and the stars. In the end, you just have to choose the best one that fits the kind of lifestyle you have and stick to it. Don't go jumping on every new diet program that launches, instead, eyes on the goal and continue on.

One of the best ways to stay on track is to practice portion control. You may exercise all you want for long periods of hours but if you eat like a Queen every single time, then you won't be able to burn all the calories you just took in. Practicing to discipline your intake will help you get slimmer faster because you're not totally eliminating your favorite treat, but rather, you're just not eating them in big chunks. While you're on this, make sure to plan your meals ahead of time so you have a proper outline on how many calories or food you're taking in. In addition, it would be best to document these somewhat like a food journal to keep track of whatever you're putting inside your mouth. Individuals who keep records are more mindful of the missteps they make and are then ready to make adjustments along the way. Food journals enable you to see your progress, both positive and negative ones. By distinguishing your unfortunate propensities, you can without much of a stretch discover substitutes for new propensities.

Stop yourself from grabbing that bag of chips. We know the temptation is so real – but hey, wouldn't it be better if you were grabbing your next pair of jeans, 3-6 sizes smaller? Don't give in to temptation. It's hard – in fact, hard is an understatement. When you're trying to lose weight, that's when all the temptations come swooping down your alley like the 4th of July. Friends suddenly invite you for drinks; family inviting you for lunch, dinner, and reunions or worse, your favorite cake just went on sale. All these, come your way when you least need them most and avoiding them will take every willpower you got. Fight it. Fight for your body, she deserves it. She has withstood all sorts of beatings emotionally, physically, and mentally and now it's time to take over. Rather than harping on the food you can't eat, attempt rather to center around what you can have. Center on it like it's the best food in the world, like you really mean how delicious it looks and tastes – you can do it.

Lastly, focus on your progress. You are beautiful in any shape, size, and form but the goal is to get healthy. So be healthy – start with the small things like skipping soda and sugary drinks to be replaced with water. Then follow off by minimizing fatty, oily food and replace them with high fiber like pineapples, watermelon, and apples. Cut yourself some slack and give yourself a good job, well done pat on the back for every small achievement. Appreciate yourself. Listen to your body. This way, you'll know when to stop and when to move forward. Recognize every accomplishment big and small. If you lost 10 lbs., celebrate with a glass of red wine. You can do it girl, you've already gone this far.

Bibliography

Adorante, M. (2017, September 28). *Why Intermittent Fasting Is the Ultimate Anti-Aging Diet*. Retrieved from W Magazine: https://www.wmagazine.com/story/why-intermittent-fasting-is-the-ultimate-anti-aging-diet

Crain, E. (2015, March 19). *15 Ways to Get Rid of Cravings in 15 Minutes or Less*. Retrieved from Women's Health Mag: https://www.womenshealthmag.com/weight-loss/g19907259/ways-to-crush-cravings/

Dr. David Jockers DC, M. C. (2016, March 8). *Benefits of Intermittent Fasting for Cancer Patients*. Retrieved from The Truth About Cancer: https://thetruthaboutcancer.com/video-benefits-of-intermittent-fasting-cancer-patients/

Frey, M. (2018, April 25). *Pros and Cons of the DASH Diet*. Retrieved from Very Well Fit: https://www.verywellfit.com/dash-diet-pros-and-cons-3973825

Kollias, H. (2018). *Intermittent Fasting for women: Important information you need to know*. Retrieved from Precision Nutrition: https://www.precisionnutrition.com/intermittent-fasting-women

Nordqvist, C. (2017, July 17). *Nine most popular diets rated by experts 2017*. Retrieved 2018, from Medical News Today: https://www.medicalnewstoday.com/articles/5847.php

Stein, N. (2017, October 03). *Pros & Cons of a Vegetarian Diet.* Retrieved from livestrong: https://www.livestrong.com/article/196211-pros-cons-of-a-vegetarian-diet/